Postinor 2

The Complete User Guide on Emergency Medication to Prevent Conception and Pregnancy

Noel James

Table of Contents

Chapter 1 3

Introduction 3

Chapter 2 8

How Does Postinor-2 Work?........................8

Chapter 3 12

Common Side Effects 12

Chapter 4 15

Dosage for Postinor-2 15

Chapter 5 19

Other Considerations for Postinor-2...........19

Chapter 6 22

Conclusion on Postinor-2 22

Chapter 1

Introduction

Postinor-2 is an emergency contraceptive pill (ECP) that is taken to prevent pregnancy within 72 hours of unprotected sex. It is a highly effective and safe form of birth control when used correctly and as directed. Postinor-2 is available in most countries around the world and is an important form of contraception for women who do not want to become pregnant and may not have access to other forms of birth control.

The active ingredient in Postinor-2 is levonorgestrel, a synthetic progestin that works by inhibiting ovulation and thickening the cervical mucus, which prevents sperm from entering the uterus. It is the most commonly used ECP and can be taken up to 72 hours (3 days) after unprotected sex.

Postinor-2 has been proven to be highly effective in preventing pregnancy when taken as directed within 72 hours of unprotected sex, with a success rate of 95%. It works best when taken as soon as possible after unprotected sex, and is more effective the sooner it is taken.

Postinor-2 is a safe and effective form of emergency contraception and should be considered an important option for women who do not want to become pregnant and may not have access to other forms of birth control. It is important to note that Postinor-2 does not protect against sexually transmitted infections and is not a substitute for regular contraception.

What is Postinor-2?

Postinor-2 is considered a highly effective method of emergency contraception, with a success rate of up to 97%. It is available in most countries with a prescription from a doctor or healthcare provider. Postinor-2 is usually taken as a single tablet, but can also be taken as two tablets 12 hours apart.

Postinor-2 is intended to be used as a backup method of contraception in cases of unprotected intercourse, contraceptive failure, or if the risk of pregnancy is high. It is not intended to be used as a primary method of birth control. It should not be used by women who are pregnant, breastfeeding, or who have recently given birth.

Postinor-2 is a safe and effective form of emergency contraception, but it is not without risks. The most common side effects are nausea, headache, and abdominal pain. Other side effects can include fatigue, breast tenderness, dizziness, and changes in menstrual bleeding. Postinor-2 may also interact with certain medications, so it is important to consult a healthcare provider before taking it.

Postinor-2 is an important option for women who have had unprotected intercourse and are at risk of pregnancy. It is important to remember that Postinor-2 is not a substitute for regular contraceptive methods and should only be used in cases of emergency.

Chapter 2

How Does Postinor-2 Work?

The active ingredient in Postinor-2 is levonorgestrel, a synthetic form of the hormone progesterone. When taken in the correct dosage, levonorgestrel prevents ovulation, or the release of an egg from the ovary, which is necessary for conception. Additionally, levonorgestrel changes the cervical mucus, making it difficult for sperm to penetrate.

Postinor-2 is most effective if taken soon after unprotected intercourse. The sooner it is taken, the more likely it will be effective in preventing pregnancy. If taken within 24 hours of unprotected intercourse, Postinor-2 is 95% effective in preventing pregnancy.

This effectiveness decreases the longer it takes to take the pill.

Postinor-2 must be taken correctly in order to be effective. It is recommended that two pills be taken as soon as possible after unprotected intercourse, with the second pill taken 12 hours after the first. Women should drink plenty of fluids while taking the pill. Additionally, women should not take more than two pills in a single cycle.

Postinor-2 is not 100% effective in preventing pregnancy and should not be used as a regular method of contraception. Additionally, Postinor-2 does not protect against sexually transmitted infections (STIs). Women should always use a barrier method of contraception, such as a condom, in addition to taking Postinor-2 if they are at risk of STIs.

Women should also be aware of the potential side effects of Postinor-2. These may include nausea, vomiting, breast tenderness, dizziness, and fatigue. If any of these side effects persist, or if any other side effects occur, women should seek medical advice.

Postinor-2 is an effective emergency contraceptive pill that can be used to prevent pregnancy after unprotected intercourse. However, it is important to remember that it is not 100% effective and should not be used as a regular method of contraception. Additionally, Postinor-2 does not protect against STIs, so a barrier method of contraception should always be used in addition to taking Postinor-2.

Chapter 3

Common Side Effects

The most common side effects of Postinor-2 are nausea and vomiting. These side effects usually occur within a few hours after taking the pill and can last for up to 24 hours. To reduce the severity of nausea and vomiting, it is recommended to take Postinor-2 with food or with an antiemetic medication such as dimenhydrinate (Dramamine).

Other common side effects of Postinor-2 include headache, dizziness, breast tenderness, abdominal pain, and changes in menstrual bleeding. These side effects are usually mild and do not require any treatment.

Severe Side Effects

Severe side effects of Postinor-2 are rare but can occur. These include allergic reactions (such as hives, difficulty breathing, and swelling of the face, lips, tongue, or throat), severe abdominal pain, and dizziness. If any of these side effects occur, it is important to seek medical attention immediately.

Risks

Postinor-2 is not recommended for women who are pregnant or breastfeeding. It is also not recommended for women who have a history of stroke, heart attack, or blood clotting disorders. It is important to discuss any potential risks with a healthcare provider before taking Postinor-2.

Conclusion

Postinor-2 is a safe and effective emergency contraceptive pill that is used to prevent pregnancy after unprotected sexual intercourse. While the side effects of Postinor-2 are generally mild, it is important to be aware of potential risks and to speak with a healthcare provider if any severe side effects occur.

Chapter 4

Dosage for Postinor-2

The recommended dose of Postinor-2 is two tablets, taken as a single dose. The tablets should be taken as soon as possible after unprotected sex, with a maximum of 72 hours. Postinor-2 can be taken with or without food.

It is important to note that Postinor-2 will not prevent pregnancy if it is taken more than 72 hours after unprotected sex. It is also important to remember that Postinor-2 does not protect against sexually transmitted infections (STIs). A barrier method of contraception such as a condom should be used to protect against STIs.

Postinor-2 is not recommended for regular use as a contraceptive. It should only be used in an emergency situation, such as after unprotected sex. If Postinor-2 is used more than once in a menstrual cycle, there is an increased risk of side effects.

If the recommended dosage is taken within the recommended time frame, Postinor-2 is 95% effective in preventing pregnancy. It is important to remember that Postinor-2 will not be effective if it is taken too late or if the dosage is not followed correctly.

It is also important to remember that Postinor-2 will not terminate an existing pregnancy. If you think you may already be pregnant, it is important to seek medical advice.

If vomiting occurs within 3 hours of taking Postinor-2, it is recommended that you take another dose. If vomiting occurs more than 3 hours after taking Postinor-2, it is not necessary to take another dose.

Postinor-2 should not be used by women who are pregnant or breastfeeding. It is also not recommended for women who are hypersensitive to any of the active ingredients in the medication.

It is important to remember that Postinor-2 is not a substitute for regular contraception. It is recommended that women use a regular method of contraception such as the pill, patch, or ring to prevent pregnancy.

If you have any questions or concerns about Postinor-2, it is important to speak to your doctor or pharmacist. They will be able to provide you with further information and advice.

Chapter 5

Other Considerations for Postinor-2

Health Considerations

Postinor-2 should not be used as a regular form of contraception, as it does not protect against sexually transmitted infections (STIs). Before taking Postinor-2, it is important to consider whether you may have been exposed to any STIs. If so, it is important to get tested and treated if necessary.

It is also important to consider any pre-existing medical conditions before taking Postinor-2. This medication can interact with certain medications, so it is important to tell your doctor about any medications or supplements you are currently taking.

Additionally, Postinor-2 may not be recommended for people with certain medical conditions, such as a history of stroke, blood clotting disorders, and some types of cancers.

Age Considerations

Postinor-2 is only approved for use by adults and adolescents over the age of 16. It is not recommended for use in children under the age of 16.

Pregnancy Considerations

Postinor-2 should not be used if you are already pregnant. It is important to take a pregnancy test before taking Postinor-2 to ensure you are not pregnant. Postinor-2 will not terminate an existing pregnancy.

Side Effects

Postinor-2 can cause some side effects, including nausea, vomiting, headaches, dizziness, fatigue, and irregular bleeding. These side effects are usually mild and should go away after a few days. If the side effects persist or become severe, it is important to contact your doctor.

It is important to consider all of these factors before taking Postinor-2. Your doctor or pharmacist can provide additional information and advice on the best contraceptive option for you.

Chapter 6

Conclusion on Postinor-2

Postinor-2 is a highly effective emergency contraceptive that can be taken up to 72 hours after unprotected intercourse or contraceptive failure. It is a safe and effective method of preventing pregnancy and is available over the counter. Postinor-2 is not suitable for regular use and should only be used in emergencies. For ongoing contraception, other methods should be discussed with a healthcare professional.

Postinor-2 has been studied extensively and has been found to be safe and effective in preventing pregnancy. It is important to remember that the earlier it is taken, the more effective it will be. The most common side effects of

Postinor-2 are nausea and vomiting, but these effects can be reduced by taking antiemetic medications.

Postinor-2 is a valuable resource for individuals who have had unprotected intercourse or contraceptive failure. It is important for individuals to understand how to use it correctly and be aware of the potential side effects. It is also important to remember that Postinor-2 should only be used in emergencies and should not be used as a regular form of contraception.

The End

www.ingramcontent.com/pod-product-compliance
Lightning Source LLC
Chambersburg PA
CBHW072347270726
48659CB00023B/2423